Health Technical Memorandum 2010

Part 1: Management policy

Sterilization

London: HMSO

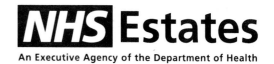

An Executive Agency of the Department of Health

ISBN 0 11 321739 0

HMSO
Standing order service

Placing a standing order with HMSO BOOKS enables a
customer to receive future titles in this series automatically
as published. This saves the time, trouble and expense of
placing individual orders and avoids the problem of
knowing when to do so. For details please write to HMSO
BOOKS (PC 13A/1), Publications Centre, PO Box 276,
London SW8 5DT quoting reference 14.02.017. The
standing order service also enables customers to receive
automatically as published all material of their choice
which additionally saves extensive catalogue research. The
scope and selectivity of the service has been extended by
new techniques, and there are more than 3,500
classifications to choose from. A special leaflet describing
the service in detail may be obtained on request.

About this publication

Health Technical Memoranda (HTMs) give comprehensive advice and guidance on the design, installation and operation of specialised building and engineering technology used in the delivery of healthcare.

They are applicable to new and existing sites, and are for use at various stages during the inception, design, construction, refurbishment and maintenance of a building.

Health Technical Memorandum 2010

HTM 2010 is being published in five parts:

this volume (Part 1) – **Management policy** – is a summary of the information required by non-technical personnel responsible for the management of sterilization services. It discusses the various types of sterilizer, for both clinical and laboratory use, and contains guidance on legal and policy matters, and on the appointment and responsibilities of personnel. It should be read by anyone consulting this memorandum for the first time;

Part 2 – **Design considerations** – contains information relevant to the specification and installation of new sterilizing equipment. It discusses the requirements for each type of sterilizer and outlines the specifications to be included in any contract. Practical considerations for the installation of sterilizers are discussed, including siting, heat emission, ventilation, noise and vibration, and mains services with an emphasis on steam quality;

Part 3 – **Validation and verification** – covers all aspects of validation and periodic testing of sterilizers. It includes detailed schedules and procedures for tests and checks to be carried out for commissioning and performance qualification, and for subsequent periodic testing;

Part 4 – **Operational management** – covers all aspects of the routine operation and maintenance of sterilizers, stressing the need for a planned maintenance programme along with the type of records to be kept. Advice on the safe and efficient operation of sterilizers is given, as well as procedures for reporting defects and accidents;

Part 5 – **Good practice guide** – provides advice on the fatigue life of pressure vessels, operational procedures guidance on the control of sterilizers, and use of the supplementary publications (logbooks etc.). It also includes a comprehensive bibliography.

The contents of this HTM in terms of management policy and operational policy are endorsed by:

a. the Welsh Office for the NHS in Wales;

b. the Health and Personal Social Services Management Executive in Northern Ireland;

c. the National Health Service in Scotland Management Executive.

References to legislation appearing in the main text of this guidance apply to the United Kingdom as a whole, except where marginal notes indicate variations for Scotland or Northern Ireland.

Contents

1.0 Sterilization and the role of management

Introduction

"The fundamental cause of this disaster is to be found in human failings ... ranging from simple carelessness to poor management of men and plant. The Committee heard of no imminent technological advance in the field of production of intravenous fluids which will eliminate the need for skilful men devoted to their work ... Too many people believe that sterilization of fluids is easily achieved with simple plant operated by men of little skill under a minimum of supervision ... Public safety in this, as in many other technological fields, depends ultimately on untiring vigilance ..."

1.1 The quotation above comes from the principal conclusions of the committee chaired by Sir Cecil Clothier and appointed to investigate an incident in which five patients died as a result of a faulty sterilizer. The tragedy led to a thorough overhaul of the methods of managing sterilizers, among which was the revision of this Health Technical Memorandum (then HTM 10), the last edition of which was published in 1980.

1.2 No disaster on a comparable scale has been reported since. Nonetheless, both the law and public opinion are now less forgiving of lapses than they were two decades ago. Tighter statutory control, resulting from new European Union (EU) Directives, will soon extend to almost every aspect of sterilization, and practices which were common a few years ago will no longer be acceptable or even lawful.

1.3 The science and art of sterilization are complex and subtle. The testing, maintenance and reporting procedures described in this HTM may seem excessive to some, but they are based upon good practice in both the UK and Europe, as formalised in European Standards designed to support the new EU Directives.

The European Union Directives on medical devices

1.4 Until now, statutory controls on the practice of sterilization, other than in the manufacture of medical products, have been few. The major Acts and Regulations which are likely to affect the management of a sterilizer are described in Chapter 3, but specific references to sterilization in the legislation are rare. This will change as a series of three EU Directives come into effect regulating the safety, quality and effectiveness of medical devices.

1.5 This section summarises basic information about the Directives. Further details are available from the Medical Devices Agency of the Department of Health.

Definition of medical device

1.6 The Directives define a medical device as any instrument, apparatus, appliance, material or other article, whether used alone or in combination, including the software necessary for its proper application intended by the manufacturer to be used on human beings for the purpose of:

a. diagnosis, prevention, monitoring, treatment or alleviation of disease;

b. diagnosis, monitoring, treatment, alleviation or compensation of an injury or handicap;

c. investigation, replacement or modification of the anatomy or of a physiological process;

d. control of conception;

and which does not achieve its principal intended action in or on the human body by pharmacological, immunological or metabolic means, but which may be assisted in its function by such means (Council Directive 93/42/EEC).

1.7   The Directives apply equally to "accessories". An accessory is defined as "an article which, whilst not being a device, is intended specifically by its manufacturers to be used together with a device to enable it to be used in accordance with the use of the device intended by the manufacturer of the device".

The three Directives

1.8   The three EU directives are as follows:

a. the Active Implantable Medical Devices Directive (Council Directive 90/385/EEC) covers all powered implants or partial implants that are left in the human body. (Heart pacemakers are the most common example of powered implants.) The directive was adopted by the EU council on 20 June 1990 and came into effect in the UK on 1 January 1993 as the Active Implantable Devices Regulations 1992 (see paragraph 3.32);

b. the Medical Devices Directive (Council Directive 93/94/EEC) covers most other medical devices ranging from first aid bandages and tongue depressors through to hip prostheses and will therefore have a wide impact on sterilization. The directive was adopted by the EU council on 14 June 1993. It will take effect on 1 January 1995, though the UK regulations have not yet been published;

c. the In-vitro Diagnostic Medical Devices Directive will cover any medical device, reagent product, kit, instrument, apparatus or system which is intended to be used in-vitro for the examination of substances derived from the human body. Some examples of in-vitro diagnostic devices are blood group reagents, pregnancy test kits, and hepatitis B test kits.

The regulatory framework

1.9   The Directives set out the essential requirements that devices must not compromise the health or safety of the patient, user or any other person and that any risks associated with the device are compatible with patient health and protection. Any side-effects must be acceptable when weighed against the intended performance.

1.10   Devices meeting these requirements will be entitled to carry the "CE" marking, signifying that the device satisfies the requirements essential for it to be fit for its intended purpose. All devices except custom-made devices and devices intended for clinical trials ("investigations" in the directive), whether used in public-sector or private-sector hospitals and nursing homes, or sold in retail outlets, will have to carry the "CE" marking.

1.11   Adoption of the Directives will mean that the UK's voluntary system of manufacturer registration and product approval for controlling certain medical devices used by the NHS will eventually be replaced by a more comprehensive statutory system covering all devices used in the UK. The Medical Devices Agency (MDA) of the Department of Health, will be the competent authority to carry out the requirements of the Directives in the UK. The main role of the MDA will ensure compliance with the UK regulations, evaluate vigilance reports received from manufacturers, and carry out a preclinical assessment of devices intended for clinical investigation. The MDA is also responsible for approving the independent certification organisations (the notified bodies) that will check and prove that defined classes of medical devices meet the essential requirements and thus enable manufacturers to apply the "CE" marking to their products.

1.12   The Medical Devices Directive includes a classification system whereby the level of regulatory control applied to devices is proportional to the degree of risk inherent in the device. The strictest controls will therefore only apply to the limited number of high-risk products.

Impact on sterilization

1.13   At the time of writing the effect of the Medical Devices Directive is being studied and will become clear when the UK regulations implementing the Directive are published. Most of the non-medical items currently processed in sterilizers are encompassed by the definition of a medical device but it is uncertain whether a sterile device emanating from, for example, a sterile services department (SSD) is to be construed as having been placed on the market by the department.

1.14   Managers who ensure that their machines and procedures comply with the guidance in this HTM should have no difficulty in complying with the Directive if and when it applies to them.

Summary of management responsibilities

1.15   HTM 2010 will assist managers and other personnel to ensure that sterilizers are operated safely and effectively and in compliance with existing and anticipated legislation and standards. To this end, the major responsibilities of management can be summarised as follows:

   a. to ensure that sterilization is carried out in compliance with the law and with the policy of the UK health departments;

   b. to ensure that all personnel connected with sterilization, whether NHS employees or contract personnel, are suitably qualified and trained for their responsibilities;

   c. to ensure that purchased sterilizers conform to legal requirements, the minimum specifications set out in British and European standards, and any additional requirements of the UK health departments;

   d. to ensure that sterilizers are installed correctly and safely with regard to proper functioning, safety of personnel and environmental protection;

   e. to ensure that newly installed sterilizers are subject to a documented scheme of validation comprising installation checks and tests, commissioning tests and performance qualification tests before they are put into service;

   f. to ensure that sterilizers are subject to a documented scheme of periodic tests at yearly, quarterly, weekly and (in some cases) daily intervals;

g.   to ensure that sterilizers are subject to a documented scheme of preventative maintenance;

h.   to ensure that procedures for production, quality control and safe working are documented and adhered to in the light of statutory requirements and accepted best practice;

j.   to ensure that procedures for dealing with malfunctions, accidents and dangerous occurrences are documented and adhered to.

2.0 Sterilizers – an overview

Introduction

2.1 This Health Technical Memorandum groups sterilizers into two broad categories according to their use:

a. **clinical sterilizers** are designed to process medical devices, medicinal products and other goods and materials that are used in the clinical care of patients;

b. **laboratory sterilizers** are designed to process goods and materials and are not directly used in the clinical care of patients.

2.2 Their operation should be kept strictly separate. Loads intended for processing in a clinical sterilizer should not be put into a laboratory sterilizer, and vice-versa.

2.3 Sterilizers can also be classified according to the sterilizing agent (the sterilant) used:

a. high-temperature steam;

b. low-temperature steam and formaldehyde;

c. ethylene oxide.

2.4 High-temperature steam is the sterilant of choice because of its superior performance. Machines using other sterilants should be reserved either for loads which would be damaged by exposure to high-temperature steam (such as certain surgical devices) or for loads that would not be sterilized by exposure to high-temperature steam (such as certain non-aqueous fluids).

2.5 Clinical sterilizers are available employing any one of the four sterilants. The laboratory sterilizers described in this HTM use only high-temperature steam.

2.6 Guidance on selection and specification, operational management, validation and verification is given in the other volumes of this HTM.

Clinical sterilizers using high-temperature steam

2.7 These are by far the most common sterilizers used in the NHS, and are manufactured in three basic types according to the nature of load they are designed to process: porous loads, fluids, or unwrapped instruments and utensils. The operating cycles are designed to cope with the differing properties of the various types of load. It is essential that a sterilizer is used only for the type of load for which it is designed.

2.8 High-temperature steam inactivates pathogens by a combination of moisture and heat. The process is well understood and the attainment of sterilization conditions can normally be confirmed by simple physical measurements. (This is not so for sterilizers using chemical sterilants, where microbiological test procedures are necessary.)

2.9 High-temperature steam sterilizers are large machines requiring permanently installed engineering services (including good-quality steam) and purpose-built accommodation. Some smaller models are transportable and generate steam from an internal reservoir.

Porous loads

2.10 Clinical sterilizers using high-temperature steam to process porous loads are commonly known as "porous load sterilizers". They are intended to deal with porous items such as towels, gowns and dressings; and medical and surgical equipment, instruments and utensils packaged or wrapped in porous materials such as paper or fabrics.

2.11 Sterilization is achieved by direct contact of the load items with good-quality saturated steam at a preferred sterilization temperature of 134°C.

2.12 As porous loads trap both air and moisture, an efficient and reliable air removal system is essential. An air detector is fitted to ensure that the operating cycle does not proceed until sufficient air and other non-condensable gases have been removed from the chamber and load. The correct functioning of the air detector is crucial to the performance of the sterilizer.

Fluids

2.13 Clinical sterilizers using high-temperature steam to process aqueous fluids are commonly known as "fluids sterilizers". They are used to sterilize fluids in sealed containers (normally bottles) of either glass or plastic. They operated at a preferred sterilization temperature of 121°C.

2.14 Fluids in glass containers can be hazardous. At a temperature of 121°C the pressure inside a one-litre bottle having a normal fill of fluid is approximately 4 bar. If the door were to be opened at this temperature, and the load exposed to ambient air, the thermal stresses arising in the glass would be sufficient to crack the bottle and cause an explosion. A temperature of 80°C is regarded as a safe maximum at which the door can be opened (even at this temperature the pressure inside a one-litre bottle is still 1.8 bar). Fluid sterilizers are fitted with a thermal door-lock to ensure that when glass containers are being processed the door cannot be opened until the temperature inside all the containers has fallen below 80°C. Failure to observe this requirement has led to serious accidents resulting from the explosion of glass containers.

2.15 Fluids in plastic containers present less of a hazard. Operating cycles for plastic containers allow the door to be opened when the temperature inside the containers falls below 90°C.

Unwrapped instruments and utensils

2.16 This type of sterilizer is used to process unwrapped surgical components intended for immediate use. Sterilization is achieved by the direct contact of the component with saturated steam at a preferred sterilization temperature of 134°C.

2.17 These sterilizers should not be used to process wrapped instruments and utensils, where the wrapping could inhibit the removal of air and the penetration of steam. Neither should they be used for unwrapped instruments and utensils with narrow lumens, where air removal and steam penetration would similarly be impaired.

2.18   Since the sterilized instruments and utensils are exposed to the air on being removed from the chamber, they are susceptible to immediate recontamination. These sterilizers are therefore suitable for clinical use only within the immediate environment in which the instruments are to be used. Wherever possible, instruments and utensils should be wrapped and processed in a porous load sterilizer.

2.19   Transportable (bench-top) models are electrically heated, requiring only a 13 A socket-outlet and no piped services. They are commonly used in theatre suites where there is no central supply service and in primary healthcare units such as general practitioners' and dentists' surgeries.

Clinical sterilizers using hot air

2.20   Clinical sterilizers using hot air as a sterilant are correctly known as "dry-heat sterilizers", and sometimes as "hot-air sterilizers" or "sterilizing ovens". They are intended to process materials such as oils, powders and some ophthalmic instruments, which can withstand high temperatures but are likely to be damaged or not sterilized by contact with steam. They operate at a preferred sterilization temperature of 160°C.

2.21   They are not suitable for use as drying cabinets (see BS2648 for specifications for drying cabinets).

2.22   Dry-heat sterilizers are essentially electric ovens and are therefore simpler than the other pressure sterilizers described in this HTM. A filter and fan are used to maintain the chamber slightly above atmospheric pressure to ensure that the sterility of the product and the integrity of the clean-room environment are not compromised. Although the cycle is under automatic control, the operator is allowed considerable freedom in selecting the required combination of sterilization temperature and time. Recommended combinations are shown in Table 2.1 and advice on their selection is given in Part 4 of this HTM (in preparation).

2.23   Dry-heat sterilizers are not efficient. It is difficult to obtain an even temperature distribution within the chamber, air circulation is inhibited when the chamber is full (even with a circulating fan), and heat transfer from the air to the load can be very slow. A complete cycle, including cooling to 80°C, takes approximately eight hours for a full test load as described in Part 3 of this HTM. If this time is unacceptable, a sterilizer fitted with assisted cooling is recommended, reducing the cycle time for the same load to approximately five hours.

Clinical sterilizers using low-temperature steam and formaldehyde

2.24   Heat-sensitive materials (wrapped or unwrapped) which will withstand saturated steam at temperatures up to 80°C are normally processed in either low-temperature steam disinfectors ("LTS disinfectors") or low-temperature steam and formaldehyde sterilizers ("LTSF sterilizers"). Sterilizers designed for LTSF will normally incorporate an LTS disinfection cycle.

2.25   Disinfection is achieved by the direct contact of the load with saturated steam at a minimum temperature of 71°C at sub-atmospheric pressure. Sterilization is achieved by contact with both saturated steam and formaldehyde gas. Either process may also be used to decontaminate soiled surgical components before they are washed and reprocessed.

2.26   Formaldehyde is a toxic gas. Part 5 of this HTM contains safety information.

2.27   Since the sterilization process is ultimately dependent on chemical action, microbiological test methods are required to confirm that sterilization conditions have been attained.

In Scotland LTSF sterilizers are considered to be disinfectors

Clinical sterilizers using ethylene oxide

2.28   Clinical sterilizers using ethylene oxide gas as a sterilant are commonly known as "ethylene oxide sterilizers" or "EO sterilizers".

2.29   EO sterilizers are used to process heat-sensitive materials and devices which cannot withstand low-temperature steam. They should not be used to process items which can be sterilized by alternative methods, that is, by high-temperature steam, dry heat or LTSF. They should not be used to re-sterilize items which have been sterilized by irradiation.

2.30   EO sterilizers are used extensively in industrial manufacture of sterile medical devices but are relatively uncommon in hospitals. Two classes of EO sterilizers are suitable for NHS use:

a.   small sterilizers, of chamber volumes around 150 litres, where the sterilant is pure EO at sub-atmospheric pressure supplied from a disposable cartridge contained within the chamber;

b.   large sterilizers, of chamber volume up to 500 litres, where the sterilant is either pure EO or EO diluted with another gas, supplied from cylinders. EO sterilizers have the potential to cause serious environmental pollution. Sterilizers using chlorofluorocarbon (CFC) gases as diluents should no longer be installed.

2.31   EO is a highly reactive liquid and gas which is toxic, flammable and explosive. The safe operation of EO sterilizers requires careful consideration of all aspects of the installation and operation of equipment.

2.32   The entire EO process is complex and requires specialised facilities for washing, packaging and preconditioning loads before processing and degassing before use. Large sterilizers will also require additional plant to dispose safely of exhaust products.

2.33   The efficacy of the process is affected by the packaging used to wrap goods for sterilization. Since the sterilization process is ultimately dependent upon chemical action, microbiological test methods are required to confirm that sterilization conditions have been attained.

2.34   Managers considering installing EO sterilizers should be aware of the following points:

a.   the difficulty in validating and monitoring suitable cleaning processes for loads before they are sterilized;

b.   the difficulty in carrying out representative performance qualification tests for the wide variety of loading conditions that may be used;

c.   the difficulty in carrying out meaningful bioburden studies on small numbers of widely differing devices to be sterilized;

d.   the problems associated with determining the levels of residual EO and its reaction products when small numbers of widely differing devices are processed.

Laboratory sterilizers/autoclaves

2.35   Laboratory sterilizers, also known as autoclaves, are used for making-safe discard material and processing apparatus and materials to be used within clinical laboratories. They are not intended for the sterilization of medical devices or medicinal products intended for the clinical care of patients.

2.36   Unlike clinical sterilizers, the laboratory sterilizers covered in this HTM are designed for use only with high-temperature steam. No chemical sterilants are used.

2.37   Certain common laboratory operations may be carried out more economically with specialised machines designed for the purpose, and these are described below.

Operating cycles

2.38   Laboratory sterilizers are often required to process a wide range of materials and objects, and they are equipped with one or more operating cycles each designed for a particular application. Different types of load generally require different operating cycles. Cycles are normally preset, and proceed automatically once selected and started.

2.39   The range of cycles that a sterilizer can provide will depend on details of its construction. For example, the methods used to remove air from the chamber, the means employed to cool and dry the load, and the provision of safety features.

2.40   Laboratory sterilizers may be equipped with one or more of the following operating cycles:

    a.   make-safe of small plastic discard;

    b.   make-safe of contained fluid discard;

    c.   sterilization of culture media;

    d.   disinfection of fabrics;

    e.   sterilization of glassware and equipment;

    f.   free steaming.

2.41   Guidance on the specification of operating cycles is given in Part 2 of this HTM.

Culture media preparator

2.42   Many of the problems which relate to sterilizing culture media can be solved by the use of small sterilizers in which the media constituents are placed directly into the chamber, thus avoiding the use of glass containers and their attendant hazards.

2.43   The machine consists of two or three modules incorporated into a system designed to provide controlled preparation, sterilization, cooling and dispensing of culture media with a minimum of attention by the operator. The system may also include a module which automatically stacks the completed culture plates.

2.44   The sterilizer module is essentially a pressure-cooker in which water and dehydrated culture media are mixed, sterilized and then cooled to below 80°C.

This type of sterilizer is particularly suitable for manufacturing batches of culture media in volumes between 1 and 20 litres.

Köch steamer

2.45   A Köch steamer is designed to expose a load to steam at near-atmospheric pressure and is commonly used for melting solidified agar. Steamers are not sterilizers and the product cannot be regarded as sterile. No further information specific to Köch steamers is given in this HTM.

Animal house sterilizer

2.46   The very wide range of materials and implements used in the care of laboratory animals is often catered for by specialised sterilizers with capacities as high as 10 m³, which run several operating cycles. Examples of loads include bedding for discard, fresh bedding, feed bottles, food and water, cages, and tools and implements for use by personnel in the animal house. In view of the specialised nature of these machines, no further information specific to animal house sterilizers is given in this HTM. Users are advised to adapt the guidance on laboratory sterilizers to their circumstances in consultation with the authorised person.

	High-temperature steam				Dry heat			LTS	LTSF	Ethylene oxide
Sterilization temperature (°C) (a)	115	121	126	134	160	170	180	71 (b)	71	30–56
Maximum allowable temperature (°C)	118	124	129	137	170	180	190	80	80	(c)
Minimum holding time (min)	30	15	10	3	120	60	30	10	180 (d)	(e)

Table 2   Sterilization temperature bands

Notes: a. The temperature setting on the automatic controller will not generally be the sterilization temperature, but a higher temperature within the sterilization temperature band.
  b. Disinfection temperature.
  c. For EO, the maximum allowable temperature will normally be 4°C above the sterilization temperature.
  d. For LTSF, the sterilization conditions may specify either a continuous holding time or the number of pulses for formaldehyde required to achieve sterilization.
  e. For EO, the "gas exposure time" is determined for each sterilizer by microbiological methods during commissioning but is typically 2–7 hours depending upon sterilization temperature and gas concentration.

3.0 Statutory requirements

Introduction

3.1 So far as sterilization is concerned, the chief areas of legislation with which managers should be familiar are health and safety, medicinal products and consumer protection.

Health and safety

The Health and Safety at Work (Northern Ireland) Order 1978 applies in Northern Ireland

3.2 The largest body of law with which managers need to be familiar concerns health and safety, in particular the Health and Safety at Work etc Act 1974 (the HSW Act) and its various regulations.

3.3 The HSW Act and its regulations require employers to assess the risk to their employees. Attention is drawn to the following hazards which are implicit in the practice of sterilization:

    a. the hazard of scalding from escaping steam;

    b. the high temperatures (up to 200°C) at which sterilizers are operated;

    c. the stored energy hazards associated with the operation of pressure vessels contained within all steam and some EO sterilizers;

    d. the stored energy hazards associated with the pressurised containers in which EO gas is transported;

    e. the explosive hazards associated with the sterilization of fluids in sealed glass bottles;

    f. the toxic properties of formaldehyde gas used in low-temperature steam and formaldehyde (LTSF) sterilizers;

    g. the toxic and explosive properties of ethylene oxide gas used in ethylene oxide (EO) sterilizers;

    h. the infection hazard associated with the microbial pathogens that may be handled by personnel using certain laboratory sterilizers;

    j. the hazard of infection to patients and staff by the inadvertent release of an unsterile load due to the failure of a sterilization and quality control process;

    k. the hazards associated with the handling of heavy and hot loads while loading and unloading sterilizers.

3.4 The guidance given throughout this HTM is designed to ensure that these hazards are minimised and that sterilization procedures comply with the relevant legislation and established good practice.

Health and Safety at Work etc Act 1974

3.5 The HSW Act sets out the basic legal responsibilities of employers and employees with regard to health and safety at work.

Management of Health and Safety at Work Regulations 1992

3.6   The Management of Health and Safety at Work Regulations 1992 (SI 1992/2051) expand upon the principles of the HSW Act.

The Management of Health and Safety at Work Regulations (Northern Ireland) 1992 apply in Northern Ireland

3.7   The core of the regulations is a requirement of employers to make a systematic assessment of the risks to health and safety of their employees and others, arising from work activities.

Workplace (Health, Safety and Welfare) Regulations 1992

3.8   The Workplace (Health, Safety and Welfare) Regulations 1992 (SI 1992/3004) aim to ensure that workplaces meet the health, safety and welfare needs of each member of the workforce, including people with disabilities.

The Workplace (Safety, Health and Welfare) Regulations (Northern Ireland) 1993 apply in Northern Ireland

3.9   Most of the regulations deal with the physical requirements of the workplace. Managers concerned with the operation of sterilizers should pay particular attention to the regulations and maintenance, ventilation, temperature, lighting, cleanliness, room dimensions and space, floors, doors and traffic routes.

Provision and Use of Work Equipment Regulations 1992

3.10   The Provision and Use of Work Equipment Regulations 1992 (SI 1992/2932) aim to ensure the provision of safe work equipment and its safe use.

The Provision and Use of Work Equipment Regulations (Northern Ireland) 1993 apply in Northern Ireland

3.11   Work equipment, defined to include "any machinery, appliance, apparatus or tool", clearly covers sterilizers and associated equipment. The requirements are numerous, and managers should ensure that all equipment first provided for use on or after 1 January 1993 complies with them. Older equipment is partly exempt until 1 January 1997.

Pressure Systems and Transportable Gas Containers Regulations 1989

3.12   The regulations on pressure systems apply to all steam sterilizers, to EO sterilizers operating above 0.5 bar, and to the steam and compressed air services. They replace the sections of the Factories Act 1961 that were relevant to steam sterilizers. The regulations on transportable gas containers apply to cartridges and cylinders used to supply sterilant or purging gas to EO sterilizers.

The Pressure Systems and Transportable Gas Containers Regulations (Northern Ireland) 1991 apply in Northern Ireland

3.13   The regulations also define the duties of the competent person: a person or organisation responsible in law for advising on the scope of a written scheme of examination of a pressure system, drawing up the scheme, certifying the scheme as being suitable, and carrying out examinations under the scheme.

NHS Estates has published a Health Guidance Note, 'The pressure systems and transportable gas containers regulations 1989', which concerns the applications of the regulation within the NHS

Control of Substances Hazardous to Health Regulations 1988

3.14   Schedule 1 of the Control of Substances Hazardous to Health (COSHH) Regulations lists ethylene oxide and formaldehyde as two substances hazardous to health which are subject to a maximum exposure limit for inhalation. These limits are reviewed annually and updated by amendments to the regulations. The current limits (1994) are given in Table 3.1. These limits must not be regarded as safe work exposures.

The Control of Substances Hazardous to Health Regulations (Northern Ireland) 1990 apply in Northern Ireland

3.15   The Health and Safety Executive (HSE) publishes an annually updated guidance note on current exposure limits – 'Occupational exposure limits (EH 40)'.

3.16   Users of laboratory sterilizers should note that a "substance hazardous to health" may include a micro-organism which creates a hazard to the health of any person. Guidance on the precautions to be taken when handling micro-organisms may be found in the Health and Safety Council (HSC) documents 'Categorisation of pathogens according to hazard and categories of containment', (second edition 1990) complied by the Advisory Committee on Dangerous Pathogens, and 'Safe working and the prevention of infection in clinical laboratories', compiled by the Health Services Advisory Committee.

Reporting of Injuries, Diseases and Dangerous Occurrences Regulations 1985

The Reporting of Injuries, Diseases and Dangerous Occurrences Regulations (Northern Ireland) 1986 apply in Northern Ireland

3.17   Commonly known as RIDDOR, these regulations impose duties on persons responsible for the activities of persons at work, and on self-employed persons, to report accidents resulting in death or major injury arising out of or in connection with work, and to report specified dangerous occurrences. They also require certain particulars of accidents at work to be reported both to the Department of Health and also to the Health and Safety Executive, and require records to be kept.

3.18   Steam and certain EO sterilizers contain pressure vessels as defined under Part 1 of Schedule 1.

3.19   Poisoning by ethylene oxide is a reportable disease listed under Schedule 2.

Manual Handling Operations Regulations 1992

The Manual Handling Operations Regulations (Northern Ireland) 1992 apply in Northern Ireland

3.20   The regulations require employers to make an ergonomic assessment of all manual handling operations which involve a risk injury, and to reduce the risk as far as is reasonably practicable. Factors to be assessed include the nature of the task, the load, the working environment and individual capability.

3.21   Managers should assess the risks associated with loading and unloading sterilizers, whether by loading trolleys or by hand. Top-loading sterilizers can be especially hazardous if lifting equipment is not available. The mass of the load is not the only source of risk; the temperature and other factors should be taken into account. Risks associated with maintenance and overhauling should also be assessed.

Personal Protective Equipment at Work Regulations 1992

The Personal Protective Equipment at Work Regulations (Northern Ireland) 1993 apply in Northern Ireland

3.22   Managers should assess whether the risks associated with sterilization require the use of personal protective equipment (PPE). Some examples include heat-resistant gloves for use when hot loads are removed from sterilizers, protective gloves for use when handling discard material in laboratories, eye or face protection when testing sterilizers containing fluids in glass bottles, and foot protection of operators loading and unloading sterilizers.

Medicinal products

Medicines Act 1968

3.23   Where a sterilizer is to be used to sterilize medicinal products, the licensing provisions of the Medicines Act 1968 apply. Further information may be found in 'Guidance to the NHS on the licensing requirements of the Medicines Act 1968', published by the Medicines Control Agency.

Medicines (Standard Provisions of Licences and Certificates) Amendment (No 3) Regulations 1977

3.24   The Medicines (Standard Provisions of Licences and Certificates) Amendments (No 3) Regulations 1977 introduced a qualified person who, in certain circumstances, has statutory responsibility for quality control in the manufacture of medicinal products (see Chapter 5). This will include decisions on release of a sterilized product.

Medicines (Standard Provision of Licences and Certificates) Amendment Regulations 1992

3.25   The Medicines (Standard Provisions of Licences and Certificates) Amendment Regulations 1992 (SI 1992/2846) give statutory force to the commission document 'The rules governing medicinal products in the European Community Volume IV: Guide to good manufacturing practice for medicinal products'. All provisions in the guide came into force on or before 1 January 1993. The annex on sterilization contains requirements that are implemented by the guidance in this HTM.

Consumer protection

3.26   In recent years, new legislation has been introduced affording protection to persons who may be harmed by unsafe goods supplied to them. In certain circumstances this may include products from sterilizers.

Consumer Protection Act 1987

3.27   Part 1 implements EU Council Directive 85/374/EEC (the Product Liability Directive) providing for compensation to be paid to persons injured by a defective product. Under the Act a product is defective "if the safety of the product is not such as persons generally are entitled to expect", taking the circumstances into account. It is likely that civil action for damages could be taken against a hospital for supplying, for example, "sterile" products that were not in fact sterile and caused the infection of a patient.

The Consumer Protection (Northern Ireland) Order 1987 applies in Northern Ireland

3.28   Part 2 introduces a "general safety requirement" on the suppliers of "consumer goods" only. It is a criminal offence to supply unsafe consumer goods, whether or not actual harm has been caused. Consumer goods are defined as "any goods which are ordinarily intended for private use or consumption", and are regarded as unsafe when "they are not reasonably safe having regard to all the circumstances". It is not clear whether products from hospital sterilizers are to be regarded as consumer goods. (Controlled drugs and licensed medicinal products are exempt from Part 2 since they are governed by other legislation.)

Electromagnetic Compatibility Regulations 1992

3.29   The Electromagnetic Compatibility Regulations (SI 1992/2372) (the EMC Regulations), impose requirements concerning the electromagnetic compatibility of most types of electrical and electronic apparatus which must be complied with, before such apparatus is to be supplied or taken into service.

3.30   A sterilizer (and any ancillary equipment) is a "relevant apparatus" within the terms of the regulations, and will have to meet standards of emission of an immunity to electromagnetic disturbance. Note that it is an offence not only to supply but also to "take into service" a sterilizer that does not conform to the regulations.

Detailed guidance on the application of the EMC regulations in healthcare premises may be found in HTM 2014 – 'Abatement of electrical interference'

3.31   The regulations do not apply to any sterilizer supplied to be taken into service in the EU before 28 October 1992. A sterilizer supplied or taken into service in the UK on or before 31 December 1995 is not required to comply with the regulations provided it complies with the requirements of the Wireless Telegraphy Acts listed in Schedule 1 of the regulations.

Active Implantable Medical Devices Regulations 1992

3.32   The Active Implantable Medical Devices Regulations 1992 (SI 1992/3146) set out the essential requirements which active implantable medical devices (such as heart pacemakers) must satisfy before they can be placed on the market or put into service.

3.33   Schedule 2, paragraph 7 requires such devices to be designed, manufactured and packed in a non-reusable packaging according to procedures which are sufficient to ensure that:

a.   the device is sterile when placed on the market; and

b.   if handled in accordance with conditions as to storage and transport laid down by the manufacturer, the device remains sterile until the packaging is removed and the device is implanted.

3.34   Schedule 2, paragraph 14 sets out requirements for the labelling of sterile packs.

Gas	Short-term exposure limits		Long-term exposure limits	
	[ppm]	[mg m^{-3}]	[ppm]	[mg m^{-3}]
Formaldehyde	2	2.5	2	2.5
Ethylene oxide	15	30	5	10

Table 3.1   Maximum exposure limits at atmospheric formaldehyde and ethylene oxide

Notes: The short-term exposure limit (STEL) is the average exposure over any 15-minute period.

The long-term exposure limit (STEL) is the exposure over any 24-hour period expressed as a single uniform exposure over an 8-hour period.

COSHH does not specify a STEL for EO. In such cases the STEL is deemed to be three times the LTEL in accordance with the recommendations of the Health and Safety Executive.

Source: HSE guidance note EH40 (1994).

4.0 British and European standards

Introduction

4.1 Industry standards for sterilization have developed rapidly since the last edition of this HTM in 1980. British standards which existed at that time have been thoroughly revised and extended. New European standards now in preparation will cover not only design, construction, performance and safety, but also validation, routine testing and operation.

4.2 British and European standards, supplemented by specific requirements for the NHS, form the basis of the guidance given in the "Design considerations" volume of this HTM.

4.3 The main standards for sterilizers are BS3970 for clinical sterilizers and BS2646 for laboratory sterilizers.

European standards

4.4 European standards on sterilization will be more extensive than British standards in specifying not only design, construction, performance and safety requirements of sterilizers, but also that persons responsible for sterilization operate a quality system and that part of that system is validation and routine testing of the process.

4.5 This edition of HTM 2010 has been written while most of the new standards are still in the course of development. While the guidance given here is designed to conform broadly with draft standards, HTM 2010 must not be regarded as a substitute for the standards themselves.

5.0 Personnel

Introduction

5.1   This chapter introduces the personnel who may share the responsibility for the safe and efficient operation of sterilizers. It gives guidance on qualifications and training and summarises areas of responsibility.

Training

5.2   It is essential that personnel at all levels have a sound general knowledge of the principles, design and functions of sterilizers. They should be trained on those types and models of sterilizers with which they are concerned. They should have some knowledge of the basic elements of microbiology in order to ensure personal safety, safety of others and general safety. Training given to individuals should be recorded and reviewed regularly.

5.3   Accredited courses on sterilization, suitable for personnel at all levels, are run at the NHS Training Centre at Eastwood Park. Further information is available from NHS Estates and the authorised persons (sterilizers).

5.4   Detailed training on particular models of sterilizer is usually available from the manufacturer, either on-site (such as during validation) or by courses at their premises.

Functional responsibility

5.5   Since the last edition of this HTM there have been profound changes in the management philosophy of the NHS. Many hospitals have become self-governing trusts, many general practices have become fund-holders, and there is a trend towards deregulation and contracting-out of services. It is not possible to prescribe a management structure of sterilization that is universally applicable given the wide range of circumstances in which a sterilizer may be employed, from a busy sterile services department in a major general hospital to a small rural dental practice.

5.6   The approach chosen for this HTM is to identify the distinct functions that need to be exercised and the responsibilities that go with them. The titles given are therefore generic; they describe the individual's role in connection with sterilization, but are not intended to be prescriptive job titles for terms of employment. Indeed, many of the personnel referred to may not be resident staff but employed by outside bodies and working on contract. Some of them will have other responsibilities unconnected with sterilization and in some cases the same individual may take on more than one role.

5.7   In every case, however, it is possible to identify a **user** who is responsible for the day-to-day management of the sterilizer. The philosophy of this HTM is to invest the user with the responsibility for seeing that the sterilizer is operated safely and efficiently.

5.8   The law requires that a **competent person (pressure vessels)** who is not the **user** is designated to exercise certain responsibilities of inspection for all steam sterilizers and other sterilizers containing pressure vessels.

5.9 For small installations where the user is qualified to perform all required test and maintenance functions, no other personnel may be necessary. This may be satisfactory for small sterilizers run by dentists or general practitioners. However, it is strongly recommended that in all cases the user receive professional advice from an **authorised person (sterilizers)**, and that testing and maintenance be carried out by a suitably qualified **test person (sterilizers)** and a **maintenance person (sterilizers)** with assistance from a **microbiologist (sterilizers)** where microbiological testing is required.

5.10 Where the sterilizer is used to manufacture medicinal products, the functions of the user are exercised by a **production manager** and a **quality controller**.

Key personnel

5.11 For the purposes of HTM 2010, the following are the key roles in the management of sterilization.

Management

5.12 Management is defined as the owner, occupier, employer, general manager, chief executive or other person who is ultimately accountable for the sole operation of its premises.

User

5.13 The user is defined as the person designated by management to be responsible for the sterilizer.

5.14 In a hospital, the user could be a sterile services department manager, laboratory manager or theatre manager; in primary care he or she could be a general practitioner, dentist, or other health professional. Where a sterilizer is used to process medicinal products, the user is normally the production manager in charge of the entire manufacturing process.

5.15 The principal responsibilities of the user are as follows:

a. to certify that the sterilizer is fit for use;

b. to hold all documentation relating to the sterilizer, including the names of other key personnel;

c. to ensure that the sterilizer is subject to periodic testing and maintenance;

d. to appoint operators where required and ensure that they are adequately trained;

e. to maintain production records;

f. to establish procedures for product release (for medical products, in cooperation with the quality controller).

Competent person (pressure vessels)

5.16 The competent person (pressure vessels) is defined as a person or organisation designated by the management to exercise certain legal responsibilities with regard to the written scheme of examination of any pressure vessel associated with a sterilizer described in the Pressure Systems and Transportable Gas Containers Regulations 1989. The shorter term "competent person" is used in this HTM.

5.17   The competent person should not be the user, nor any of the other key personnel associated with the sterilizer in question.

5.18   The following guidance on the qualifications of the competent person is based on the HSC Approved Code of Practice 'Safety of pressure systems':

a.   where required to draw up or certify schemes of examination, the competent person should be qualified at least to technician engineer level, with adequate relevant experience and knowledge of the law, codes of practice, examination and inspection techniques and understanding of the effects of operation for the pressure vessel concerned. He or she must have established access to basic design and plant operation advice, materials engineering and non-destructive testing facilities. The competent person must have sufficient organisation to ensure a reasonable data storage and retrieval system with ready access to relevant law, technical standards and codes;

b.   where required to carry out examinations, the competent person should have sufficient practical and theoretical knowledge and actual experience of the type of pressure vessel which is to be examined to enable defects or weaknesses to be detected and their importance in relation to the integrity and safety of the sterilizer to be assessed.

5.19   The principal duties of the competent person under the regulations are as follows (they need not all be exercised by the same individual):

a.   advising on the scope of the written scheme of examination;

b.   drawing up the written scheme of examination or certifying the scheme as being suitable;

c.   carrying out examinations in accordance with the written scheme, assessing the results and reviewing the written scheme for its suitability.

5.20   Most insurance companies maintain a technical division able to advise on appointing a competent person. The authorised person (sterilizers) will also be able to provide advice.

5.21   Further information about the written scheme of examination will be found in Part 4 of this HTM.

Authorised person (sterilizers)

5.22   The authorised person (sterilizers) is defined as a person designated by management to provide independent auditing and advice on sterilizers and sterilization and to review and witness documentation on validation. The shorter term "authorised person" is used in this HTM.

5.23   The authorised person should:

a.   have a minimum of two years' recent experience in the validation of sterilization processes to modern standards;

b.   have a degree in a relevant science subject or corporate membership of a relevant professional institution;

c.   have completed an accredited course for authorised persons (sterilizers) and successfully passed the examination;

or alternatively, should:

d.   have applied for registration as an authorised person (sterilizers) no later than 31 December 1994;

    e. have at least ten years' experience in the validation of porous load and laboratory sterilization processes;

    f. have two years' experience in a responsible position;

    g. successfully pass an accredited examination for authorised persons (sterilizers) within five years of registration.

5.24 The authorised person is required to liaise closely with other professionals in various disciplines and consequently, the appointment should be made known in writing to all interested parties. He or she should have direct contact with the user and other key personnel.

5.25 The principal responsibilities of the authorised person are as follows:

    a. to provide general and impartial advice on all matters concerned with sterilization;

    b. to advise on programmes of validation;

    c. to audit reports on validation, revalidation and yearly tests prepared by the test person;

    d. to advise on programmes of periodic tests and periodic maintenance;

    e. to advise on operational procedures for routine production.

5.26 A register of suitably qualified authorised persons is maintained by the Institution of Hospital Engineering.

Test person (sterilizers)

5.27 The test person (sterilizers) is defined as a person designated by management to carry out validation and periodic testing of sterilizers. The shorter term "test person" is used in this HTM.

5.28 The test person should:

    a. be qualified to at least HNC in engineering or microbiological sciences;

    b. have completed an accredited course for test persons (sterilizers) and successfully passed the examination;

    c. have been recently employed in an NHS hospital with responsibility for validation and periodic testing for one or more sterilization processes;

or alternatively:

    d. have a certificate demonstrating satisfactory completion of an accredited course (City and Guilds or equivalent) in the validation and periodic testing of at least two sterilization processes;

    e. have at least three years' experience in the validation and periodic testing of porous load sterilizers and at least one other sterilization process.

5.29 The principal responsibilities of the test person are as follows:

    a. to conduct the validation tests specified in Part 3 of this HTM and to prepare the validation report;

    b. to conduct the periodic tests specified in Part 3 and to prepare reports as required by the user;

    c. to conduct any additional tests at the request of the user.

Maintenance person (sterilizers)

5.30   The maintenance person (sterilizers) is defined as a person designated by management to carry out maintenance duties on sterilizers. The shorter term "maintenance person" is used in this HTM.

5.31   The maintenance person should be a fitter or an electrician with documentary evidence to demonstrate competence in the maintenance of one or more types of sterilizer. He or she should be in a position to deal with any breakdown in an emergency and have the ability to diagnose faults and carry out repairs or to arrange for repairs to be carried out by others.

5.32   The principal responsibilities of the maintenance person are as follows:

  a. to carry out the maintenance tasks outlined in Part 4;

  b. to carry out additional maintenance and repair work at the request of the user.

5.33   A maintenance person who has a minimum of two years' experience in the maintenance of sterilizers and who has obtained a recognised qualification in the testing of sterilizers may perform the duties of the test person for the daily, weekly and quarterly tests described in Part 3.

Microbiologist (sterilizers)

5.34   The microbiologist (sterilizers) is defined as a person designated by management to be responsible for advising the user on microbiological aspects of the sterilization of non-medical products. The shorter term "microbiologist" is used in this HTM.

5.35   The microbiologist should have a relevant degree (for example microbiology or medicine) and will normally be a member of the hospital staff.

5.36   The principal responsibilities of the microbiologist are as follows:

  a. to advise the user on the microbiological aspects of sterilization procedures for non-medicinal products;

  b. to arrange for the culturing of biological indicators used in microbiological tests (normally low-temperature steam and formaldehyde (LTSF) and ethylene oxide (EO) sterilizers);

  c. to audit the documentation from all sterilizers which have been tested by microbiological methods.

Personnel for medicinal products

5.37   Where a sterilizer is to be used in the production of medicinal products, the provisions of the Medicines Act 1968 apply. The responsibilities that would otherwise be exercised by the user are divided between the production manager and the quality controller. Guidance on the duties of each can be found in the EU commission document 'Guide to good manufacturing practice for medicinal products'.

Production manager

5.38   The production manager is defined as a person designated by management to be responsible for the production of medicinal products.

Quality controller

5.39   The quality controller is defined as a person designated by management to be responsible for quality control and medicinal products with authority to establish, verify and implement all quality control and quality assurance procedures.

5.40   He or she should have the authority, independent of the production manager, to approve materials and products and to reject, as seen fit, raw materials, packaging materials, and intermediate, bulk and finished products not complying with the relevant specification or not manufactured in accordance with approved procedures.

5.41   The quality controller should be professionally qualified (for example in pharmacy). Any additional qualifications will depend on the type of licence which is held, for example:

a. where a product licence is held, the quality controller should satisfy the requirements of the qualified person as defined in the Medicines (Standard Provisions of Licences and Certificates) Amendment (No. 3) Regulations 1977. If the quality controller does not meet these requirements, a qualified person should be designated to exercise the functions specified in the regulations;

b. where the manufacturer's licence "specials" is held, as is generally the case in hospitals, the quality controller need not satisfy the requirements of a qualified person.

5.42   Further information about qualified person can be found in MAL 45 Medicines Acts 1968, 1971.

Other personnel

5.43   The following personnel are also mentioned in this HTM.

5.44   The **laboratory safety officer** is defined as a person designated by management to be responsible for all aspects of laboratory safety including equipment, personnel and training relating to safety issues, and ensuring compliance with safety legislation and guidelines.

5.45   An **operator** is defined as any person with the authority to operate a sterilizer, including the noting of sterilizer instrument readings and simple housekeeping duties.

5.46   The **manufacturer** is defined as a person or organisation responsible for the manufacturer of a sterilizer.

5.47   The **contractor** is defined as a person or organisation designated by management to be responsible for the supply and installation of the sterilizer, and for the conduct of the installation checks and tests. The contractor is commonly the manufacturer of the sterilizer.

Other publications in this series

(Given below are details of all Health Technical Memoranda available from HMSO. HTMs marked (*) are currently being revised, those marked (†) are out of print. Some HTMs in preparation at the time of publication of this HTM are also listed.)

1 Anti-static precautions: rubber, plastics and fabrics*†

2 Anti-static precautions: flooring in anaesthetising areas (and data processing rooms)*, 1977.

3 –

4 –

5 Steam boiler plant instrumentation†

7 Protection of condensate systems: filming amines†

2007 Electrical services: supply and distribution, 1993.

8 –

9 –

2011 Emergency electrical services, 1993.

12 –

13 –

2014 Abatement of electrical interference, 1993.

2015 Bedhead services, 1994.

16 –

17 Health building engineering installations: commissioning and associated activities, 1978.

18 Facsimile telegraphy: possible applications in DGHs†

19 Facsimile telegraphy: the transmission of pathology reports within a hospital – a case study†

2020 Electrical safety code for low voltage systems, 1993.

2021 Electrical safety code for high voltage systems, 1993.

2022 Medical gas pipeline systems, 1994.

23 Access and accommodation for engineering services†

24 –

2025 Ventilation in healthcare premises, 1994.

26 Commissioning of oil, gas and dual fired boilers: with notes on design, operation and maintenance†

27 Cold water supply storage and mains distribution* [Revised version will deal with water storage and distribution], 1978.

28 to 39 –

2040 The control of legionellae in healthcare premises – a code of practice, 1993.

41 to 49 –

2050 Risk management in the NHS estate, 1994.

51 to 54 –

2055 Telecommunications (telephone exchanges), 1994.

Component Data Base (HTMs 54 to 70)

54.1 User manual, 1993.

55 Windows, 1989.

56 Partitions, 1989.

57 Internal glazing, 1989.

58 Internal doorsets, 1989.

59 Ironmongery, 1989.

60 Ceilings, 1989.

61 Flooring, 1989.

62 Demountable storage systems, 1989.

63 Fitted storage systems, 1989.

64 Sanitary assemblies, 1989.

65 Signs†

66 Cubicle curtain track, 1989.

67 Laboratory fitting-out system, 1993.

68 Ducts and panel assemblies, 1993.

69 Protection, 1993.

70 Fixings, 1993.

71 to 80 –

Firecode

81 Firecode: fire precautions in new hospitals, 1987.

81 Supp 1 1993.

82 Firecode: alarm and detection systems, 1989.

83 Fire safety in healthcare premises: general fire precautions, 1994.

85 Firecode: fire precautions in existing hospitals, 1994.

86 Firecode: fire risk assessment in hospitals, 1994.

87 Firecode: textiles and furniture, 1993.

88 Fire safety in health care premises: guide to fire precautions in NHS housing in the community for mentally handicapped/ill people, 1986.

New HTMs in preparation

Lifts
Combined heat and power
Washers for sterile production

Health Technical Memoranda published by HMSO can be purchased from HMSO bookshops in London (post orders to PO Box 276, SW8 5DT), Edinburgh, Belfast, Manchester, Birmingham and Bristol, or through good booksellers. HMSO provide a copy service for publications which are out of print; and a standing order service.

Enquiries about Health Technical Memoranda (but not orders) should be addressed to: NHS Estates, Department of Health, Marketing and Publications Unit, 1 Trevelyan Square, Boar Lane, Leeds LS1 6AE.

About NHS Estates

NHS Estates is an Executive Agency of the Department of Health and is involved with all aspects of health estate management, development and maintenance. The Agency has a dynamic fund of knowledge which it has acquired during 30 years of working in the field. Using this knowledge NHS Estates has developed products which are unique in range and depth. These are described below.

NHS Estates also makes its experience available to the field through its consultancy services.

Enquiries should be addressed to: NHS Estates, 1 Trevelyan Square, Boar Lane, Leeds LS1 6AE. Tel: 0532 547000.

Some other NHS Estates products

Activity DataBase – a computerised system for defining the activities which have to be accommodated in spaces within health buildings. *NHS Estates*

Design Guides – complementary to Health Building Notes, Design Guides provide advice for planners and designers about subjects not appropriate to the Health Building Notes series. *HMSO*

Estatecode – user manual for managing a health estate. Includes a recommended methodology for property appraisal and provides a basis for integration of the estate into corporate business planning. *HMSO*

Capricode – a framework for the efficient management of capital projects from inception to completion. *HMSO*

Concode – outlines proven methods of selecting contracts and commissioning consultants. It reflects official policy on contract procedures. *HMSO*

Works Information Management System – a computerised information system for estate management tasks, enabling tangible assets to be put into the context of servicing requirements. *NHS Estates*

Health Building Notes – advice for project teams procuring new buildings and adapting or extending existing buildings. *HMSO*

Health Facilities Notes – debate current and topical issues of concern across all areas of healthcare provision. *HMSO*

Health Guidance Notes – an occasional series of publications which respond to changes in Department of Health policy or reflect changing NHS operational management. Each deals with a specific topic and is complementary to a related Health Technical Memorandum. *HMSO*

Encode – shows how to plan and implement a policy of energy efficiency in a building. *HMSO*

Firecode – for policy, technical guidance and specialist aspects of fire precautions. *HMSO*

Concise – software support for managing the capital programme. Compatible with Capricode. *NHS Estates*

Model Engineering Specifications – comprehensive advice used in briefing consultants, contractors and suppliers of healthcare engineering services to meet Departmental policy and best practice guidance. *NHS Estates*

Items noted "HMSO" can be purchased from HMSO Bookshops in London (post orders to PO Box 276, SW8 5DT), Edinburgh, Belfast, Manchester, Birmingham and Bristol or through good booksellers.

Enquiries about NHS Estates should be addressed to: NHS Estates, Marketing and Publications Unit, Department of Health, 1 Trevelyan Square, Boar Lane, Leeds LS1 6AE.

NHS Estates consultancy service

Designed to meet a range of needs from advice on the oversight of estates management functions to a much fuller collaboration for particularly innovative or exemplary projects.

Enquiries should be addressed to: NHS Estates, Consultancy Service (address as above).

Printed in the United Kingdom for HMSO
Dd296836 3/94 C14 G3396 10170